# Mushrooms:

## Learn How to Identify, Harvest And Preserve Medicinal Mushrooms

# Table of Contents

## Introduction

Welcome to Medicinal Mushrooms, a D.I.Y. book about navigating the fields of mushrooms in order to get the medicinal benefits that mushrooms can provide. This book takes the art of mushroom picking very seriously because while mushrooms are currently at the forefront of some pharmaceutical industries for helping to cure the sick, they are also very well known for having unintended effects, which including being high and dying. Talk about your lows and highs in the Mushroom Kingdom. With that said, let's begin.

# Chapter 1 – A Word of Warning and The Medical Properties You Need

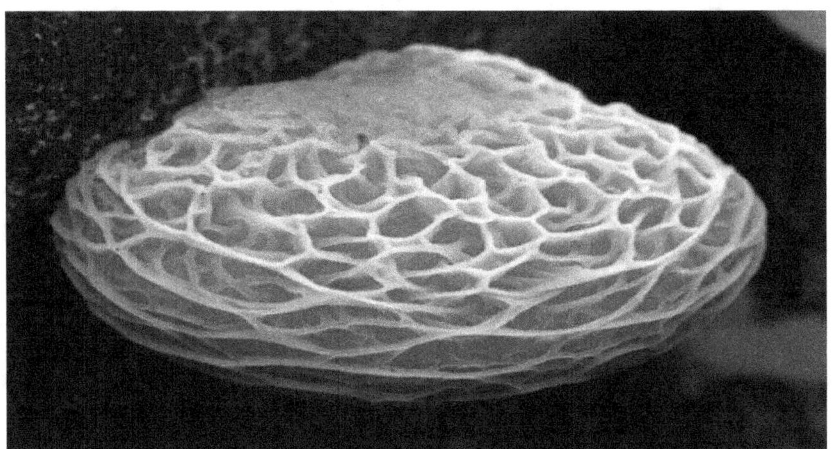

Now, a lot of people think of mushrooms and automatically think either it's a wonderful healing object or that it is an object of massive hallucinations that one will either love or fear for the rest of their life. The truth is that it's a little bit of a mixture of all of this depending on which family of mushroom you choose. This is because mushrooms have developed certain tendencies towards defending themselves and all of the methods that you describe provide a method of healing itself or defending itself.

### *Fear The Unknown*

Let me take you on a story of a man who's desperate for food. The man hasn't eaten in a couple of days and his entire body aches because of the lack of food. However, the man believes he has a firm understanding of what fungus can kill him and what fungus can't kill him so he happens upon a field of mushrooms that look absolutely divine. He picks up a couple of mushrooms and brings them back to the camp with them. He plucks them inside of a camping pot that he boils in order to make mushroom soup or at least the most basic form of mushroom soup as we can possibly think it will be. This soup is ready in about an hour or two and he could sip it down with delight.   As he heads off to bed and he says his goodnights to whatever person he might, this is the last time he will wake up because he didn't notice that the mushrooms he picked put white fluid on his hands. This represents one of the most poisonous types of mushrooms on the planet and it is extremely easy to miss if you're in a bad shape.

It's very important that you realize that mushrooms can either save you, heal you or kill you but never just two or all three. Unless you are 100% positive that the mushroom in front of you is non-toxic and will benefit you, along with experience from picking that same type of mushroom in comparison to the toxic mushrooms it can be compared with, do not ever touch a mushroom if you do not know what it is. There are tons, possibly hundreds, of possible toxin mushrooms in the wild and they will drop you without any sign of being poisoned. I know that this sounds like an apocalypse prophecy but it is true and it has happened quite often. There's a reason why this is a movie trope in Hollywood. With that said, with plenty of practice and skill you can usually bend mushrooms to your advantage if you really need to. Additionally, you don't need to know whether a mushroom is poisonous or not if you're buying from a trusted seller and I don't mean the guy who happens to have some mushrooms down the streets that he thinks will be excellent for you, stay away from that guy. Instead, I'm talking about the stores like GNC or Nutrition Plus, someone you can sue if you happen to get sick from eating a type of mushroom.


Most of the mushrooms that you will be dealing with that could be toxic are usually very noticeable in their toxicity. For example, leaving white viscous fluid on your hand is a very noticeable thing if you're not dehydrated and lacking food over several days, which can normally get you killed in any other way as well as mushroom poisoning. However, there are a few mushrooms that look absolutely harmless but will kill you and these are mushrooms that you need to really look out for and compare them to mushrooms that you already know of. This guide will go over the different type of mushrooms that there are that are medicinally available to you but this guide is not going to help you identify those types of mushroom. Instead, I highly encourage you to go to a mushroom farm or go to a mushroom grower and learn from them rather than from a book that will have no pictures of mushrooms. Mushrooms are something you need to identify through look, smell, touch, and, even, taste sometimes. However, if you are the type of person in which you do not need to know what the mushrooms look like and you just want to know the ones that are medicinal so you can buy them at the store, this is going to be the longest collection of medicinal herbs that you can possibly buy in an online store or an offline store. Let's go over some of the awesome properties of what some of these fungi are capable of doing.

### *Popular Properties*

- Antibacterial

A lot of people don't realize that penicillin is an actual type of fungus and that the antibiotics that we get today mostly come from mushrooms. In an ironic twist, the most notable fungi for producing antibacterial properties is the penicillium mold otherwise known as penicillin. However, mold is not the same as a mushroom and the mushrooms that we tend to get antibiotics from are the ones that metabolite pleuromutilin. Just so you know, we will not be getting into heavy amounts of medicinal reading material because this is not a medicine academy.

- Cholesterol

Some of the very first cholesterol inhibitors came from fungus. However, this came from an unexpected source that we only considered useful to be an antibiotic; penicillium. While most of these are now made from forms of yeast, that does not mean that mushrooms do not help lower cholesterol. It is just that mushrooms are less effective than yeast.

- Fungus can be Antifungal?

While it may be shocking to hear at first, it isn't surprising once you realize that it is a matter of defense. Some mushrooms have had to deal with other families of mushrooms and an order to deal with that family of mushrooms they had to develop properties that could naturally fight that type of mushroom. This means that some fungus have antifungal properties.

- Malaria

As of right now, there are about 4 different fungi that are  used to treat malaria. However, these are often extracted inside of a laboratory and will not be useful to the average individual.

- Immunosuppressant

Cyclosporin, Bredinin, and Mycophenolic acid are some of the common ones that were given to use via a fungal family.

- Vitamins

Almost all mushrooms are capable of giving you a very specific vitamin called vitamin D and this is good for your bones along with several other different factors. Fungus, in particular, are really good at synthesizing vitamin D.

## Chapter 2 – Understanding Mushroom Family Trees

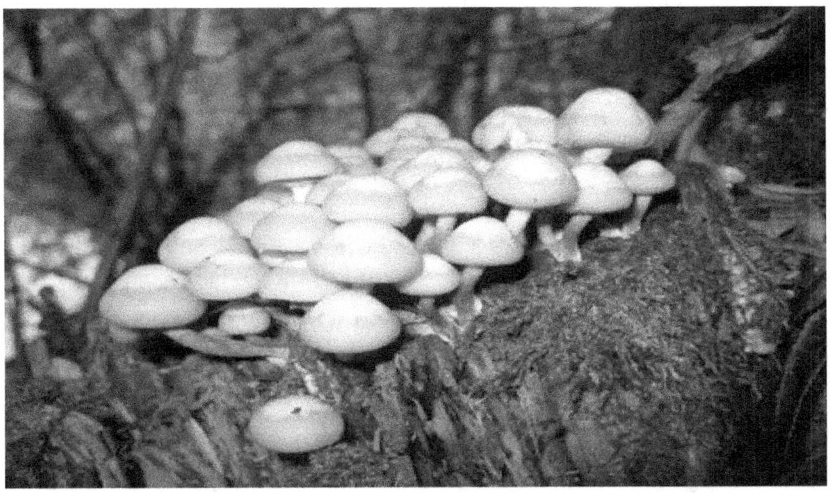

Whenever you hear gardeners talk about their mushrooms or herbalists talk about mushroom plant effects, they also tend to say the mushroom family or the mushroom genus. The reason for this is that mushrooms are kind of like humans in the fact that most of the mushrooms that you see are different from other mushrooms that you see even though they have the same name of family. Mushrooms that grow separate from each other may stem from the same genetic material but their environment changes how they actually deal with their development. An example of how this change could occur is if a mushroom is in a desert rather than a forest and they need to protect themselves from the local environment of heat rather than any potential vegetarian animals out there otherwise known as herbivores for those that do not know.  Now, if you took that same mushroom plant and transported it into a livable area for the mushroom but it was full of forestry then, given another hundred or two hundred years, you would see a slow transformation of different attributes in comparison to its desert family brethren. This is because the 2 mushrooms have had to deal with different circumstances and, therefore, even though they are technically from the same root plant, they did have to develop different traits in comparison.

The reason why I'm bringing this up is because when we talk about the potential health effects of a certain type of plant, especially mushrooms, we also have to realize that some of the family don't have access to those same benefits. For instance, an anti-inflammatory benefit could arise in one plant that needed it in order to deal with the pain of the atmosphere whereas another plant didn't really need it because the environment wasn't that painful. I'm not saying that plants develop the anti-inflammatory trait because they're in pain but the example shows you how they might have one benefit over another and this is what makes it difficult to say which mushrooms are the best mushrooms of the family to give you medicinal benefits.

### *Where are Most Mushrooms?*

Now, while some variations of mushrooms tend to hide in different types of places than one would normally expect them, the most common place to find mushrooms is where there is life. Most fungi are parasitic plants and the fact that they feed off of either the dead organisms that fell to the ground or even the live organisms is the key factor to most mushrooms as they are very close to a highly organic source in order to allow them to grow exponentially. If mushrooms are not able to grow at a very quick rate than they usually die from lack of growth. This is one of the oddest things to see in a plant because most plants will take a certain amount of time in order to grow and tend to only suffer from overcrowding.

The reason why its parasitic is because mushrooms will usually kill the soil that it is inside of in order to continuously expand its network. Mushrooms tend to have a very good network of plant communications because mushrooms are very low to the ground and they are a type of parasite rather than just a plant that grows out of the ground, which means they could be seen as a continuous source of food if they are not aggressive. They need this type of network in order to expand and spread their seeds to more areas where they can suck up more sources of organisms. With that said, the soil where mushrooms die at is usually extremely fertile once the mushroom has fully decayed into it because mushrooms withhold a lot of moisture inside of those gills and the entire bulb and stem is full of nutrients that most plants would not condense inside of the stem. As I said, there are few different mushrooms that are a little bit weird, but the most common types of mushrooms will be found at either the base of a tree, on a dead organism, on the sides of a tree, or in a very dense and damp area where there is a lot of water along with a lot of nutrients.

## Chapter 3 – The Poison Test

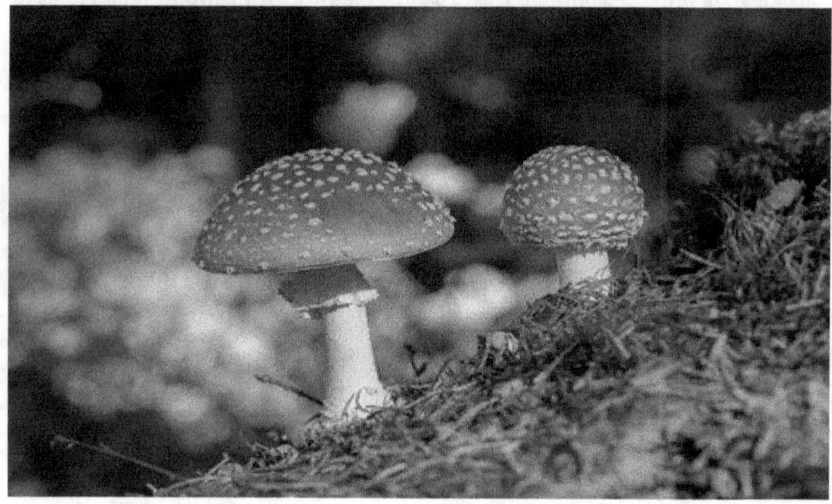

Even though the main advice from most herbalist is to just avoid ever having to deal with a poisonous mushroom by not ingesting the one that you are not completely sure about, there are some ways to identify the more obviously poisonous ones. I'm going to go ahead and tell you these because if you become experienced with picking your own mushrooms than these might come in handy, but that doesn't mean they're always going to work for you because the obvious ones are protecting themselves from being eaten whereas the line obvious ones are trying to remove the threat from its surrounding plants. It's kind of like the suicidal kamikaze that used to kill themselves in order to deal the most damage to their enemies. Only, this is the fungus trying to kill you before you eat any of its brethren in the future.

*How much do you need to worry?*

I probably scared most of the people who aren't familiar with the mushroom and how deadly it can be but it is truly vital that you understand how easy it is to mess up on what you're trying to pull out of the ground. Take the chestnut mushroom, which is one of the medicinal plants that we're going to talk about in the section where I list the top medicinal. It is suggested by almost every single professional that unless you are, in fact, a professional yourself, with years of study in mushrooms, that you do not try to figure out if a chestnut mushroom is going to kill you or if it's going to give you medicine that you're looking for. The reason for this is because almost all chestnut mushrooms look identical to most people and there are small subtle differences between the variations of chestnut mushrooms that are beneficial to you vs. the variations of chestnut mushrooms that have developed a toxicity to them. There are a few ways to determine if something is poisonous and these are ways that you can use if you're in an absolute dire situation, but the problem with this is that it's not one hundred percent accurate. There are some poisons that take days to show up and these types of poisons can easily just walk right past some of these circumstances used in order to detect whether something is poisonous or not. Additionally, if something isn't poisonous in small amounts then you likely won't feel anything, much like the cyanide inside of apple seeds. If you eat one or two seeds of the apple seed then you are likely not going to experience a death by cyanide but if you were to have around 500 to 1000 of the seeds at once, I don't know why you would do this but you would experience cyanide death. This is why it is important to not only know which  plants you are pulling out of the ground but that you know every single part of the plant and that you've memorized it, studied it, and make sure that you know exactly what you are doing.

### *The Common Poisonous Traits*

There are a few traits that you need to pay attention to in order to identify most of the poisonous mushrooms that are out there. The first thing that you need to pay attention to is the color and where it is at and the two colors you need to specifically notice are the white and red colors. If the red is on the cap or on the stem then you most likely want to avoid that as that usually means it is poisonous. If it's got something like white gills, or a skirt, or a ring on the actual stem and then is automatically accompanied by a sack, known as a vulva, then you don't really want to test your luck with this type of plant. An example of a family that usually just exudes the toxicity examples that we've explained here would be the milk caps family and that is because almost all of them have the white gills that we were talking about and the white viscous fluid that would go on your hand as I was talking about that before. Mushrooms are not supposed to leak liquid, just so you know. Another common test that you can sometimes use on certain mushrooms, provided that you know enough to avoid the blatantly obvious poisonous ones, is a taste test. Most of the poisonous ones are usually very bitter to the taste because they don't want you to be eating them. I guess the poison that comes afterwards if you do decide to eat it is just punishment that you were asking for. Just saying, you know, there are about 7,000 cases of people eating poisonous mushrooms a year and usually a much smaller amount of deaths that result from that because of the wonderful work that hospitals do to save us from our stupid decisions.


The true problem with poisonous plants is that sometimes they don't follow the guidelines that we've shown you here and these tend to be the most deadly ones because people tend to fall into their trap easier. Take the chestnut for example, which is a plant that is usually very easily identifiable and has a lot more non-deadly/nontoxic versions of it in comparison to the toxic versions. This large ratio difference caused a lot of people who are used to using Chestnut mushrooms in their soups or in their teas to be poisoned by the mushroom simply because they didn't know that there existed a poisonous version of it. If you're in an unknown area that not many people travel in then you have a much higher chance of discovering a type of mushroom that no one has classified yet and this is where you come into contact with the most amount of issues if you are a professional. Knowing your family is really important in the Mushroom Kingdom and if you don't know a certain mushroom then just leave it alone unless you are in a situation where dying is where you are either are going to die from not eating it or you're going to die from eating it. Unless you're in that type of situation, I don't suggest you ever try any mushroom that you  don't have a 100% clearing of your knowledge to say that that mushroom is not poisonous.

### *The Poison Test*

There's a poison test that you can do with pretty much any type of plant that you want to see if it's poisonous or not and this is for those who are in immediate need for nutritional value because otherwise they're going to die. What I mean by immediate need is that you need about two to three days for you to be able to test whether the food in front of you is poisonous or not and even then it's not a guarantee. You first begin by placing whatever it is on your arm, your leg or any other spot that you don't mind having a rash at but that you remember where you used it so that you can tell whether the plant is poisonous not. You rub it on your skin and then you wait 24 hours to see if anything happen. Then you place it on your tongue and take out off immediately and then wait another 24 hours to see if anything happened. Finally, you place it on your tongue and leave it there for at least 30 seconds and then you take it off and you wait 24 hours to see if anything happens. There is a potential final step and that's where you just eat off a very tiny portion of the food and then wait 24 hours to see if anything happens. However, some plants can kill you with this small amount of food so that isn't really a viable option in some circumstances. With that said, this will generally get rid of the most poisonous plants that you'll come up against but some of the more sneaky ones will be able to get past this  detection method.


The reason why this works is because poison will usually attack anything that it comes in contact with regardless of what it is attacking. This means that the skin that it is attacking is being attacked by the irritants of the poisonous material. Then you have the fact that your tongue absorbs a small portion of the poison and will provide you with adverse effects if the material is poisonous. This is a dangerous step because some materials can be so poisonous that just putting it on your tongue can kill you but these are very rare. The same can be said of putting it on your skin because there are even some mushrooms that are so deadly that if you put it on your skin and wait a little while you can usually see if it will kill you. The most advanced form of this is if you take a small bite of it and wait to see what happens because then the more sneaky ones come out and decide to attack your system. Most poisons will activate within the first 24 hours but there were a few on this planet that take days in order for it to happen. This can be a very unreliable test in some circumstances but in most circumstances it can help you get out of a really bad situation provided that the only way that you were going to get out of the situation was if you were going to die. That's a really bleak view on a method that supposed to help you survive.

# Chapter 4 – Top Medicinal Mushrooms

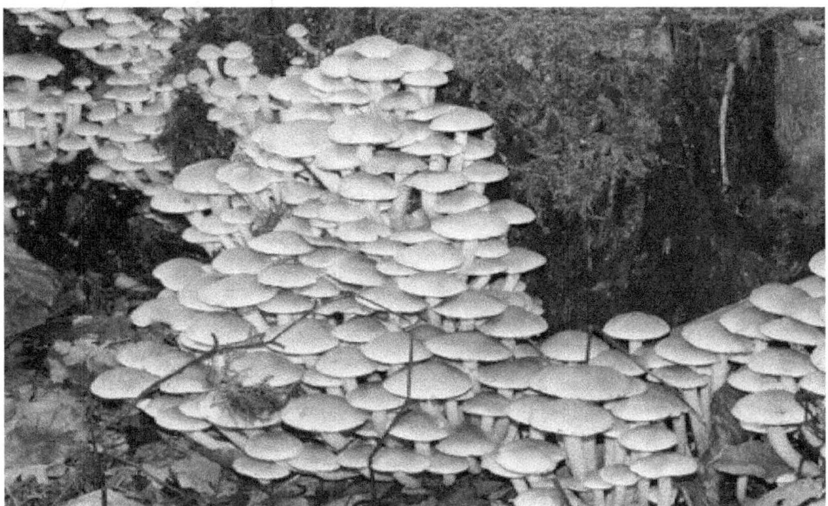

*Mushrooms - All Climates*

Reishi

The Reishi mushroom is good for mostly cancer treatment but also dealing with high blood pressure and cholesterol. Most notably this mushroom is really good at handling ovarian  cancer but scientists don't know yet which stage this mushroom would be best use that. The way it fights cancer is it basically just stops new cells from fully forming.

Shiitake

This mushroom is also good for cancer treatment and works a lot like the previous mushroom that we just talked about. It's also really high in potassium, niacin, calcium, magnesium, phosphorus and B vitamins. It is already being used to fight stomach cancer.

Tinder Conk

This mushroom is mostly an anti-infective and some surgeons have used this to stop the bleeding. a dentist who is been out of practice for a few years may use this in order to stop the bleeding if they're doing any type of dental work because this was a common practice. however just because doctors tend to use it to help treat infections it is also still really useful in the treatment for throat cancer as well as cancer of the uterus.

God's Mushroom

Even though the name suggests that it might be the all mighty powerful mushroom it is clearly not in comparison to the ones we've seen before. While it is good and help being alleviate some of the issues with two types of cancers, most of the time this mushroom will inhibit cancer growth. Beyond that, it is really good for handling insulin and blood sugar levels and side of people as well as being in general immune system booster.

Common Mushroom

While the name may be a misnomer, the common mushroom is more or less the commoner of mushrooms. It doesn't really specialize in any one thing and it doesn't really do any one thing particularly well. What it does do is help prevent diseases from occurring in the first place, a lot like green tea does. For instance, a study was done to show that it helped decrease the risk for cancer inside of the breast by nearly 90%. Beyond that, the mushroom doesn't really have that many medicinal properties worth of value. Additionally, the mushroom is full of potassium which can be detrimental to your health if you consume too much of it like you would if you were to take it as a medicine.

### Mushrooms - Cold Climates 40- Deg F

Maitake

This mushroom is like the cure-all mushroom because it fights cancer, boost the immune system, helps control blood sugar and cholesterol, and even helps you lose weight. The particular type of cancer that it fights is breast cancer and the second part that it does is it helps alleviate some of the issues that people suffering from type 2 diabetes have to deal with on a daily basis, which comes in the form of helping to increase insulin sensitivity.

Chaga

The chaga specializes in a lot of the more rare types of treated illnesses. This mushroom is really good for helping out with psoriasis, tuberculosis, and gastritis. In a study done in Russia, they treated psoriasis patients with chaga and found that the patient's completely recovered.

Birch Bracket

This mushroom mainly serves as a mushroom containing anti-inflammatory properties and can be used as both an antibiotic and an antiviral. Additionally, almost like any other of the mushrooms found on the list it can fight a general wide category of different cancers but has specifically showing that it's really good at fighting Sarcoma 180 and Ehrlich solid cancers by nearly 90%.

### *Mushrooms - Hot Climates 60+ Deg F*

Oyster

This mushroom is really good at fighting high levels of cholesterol by balancing out the HDL and the LDL and is also really good at fighting bacteria, which means that it's a good antibiotic to have. Otherwise, the mushroom doesn't really do much beyond that.

Lion's Mane

This mushroom is really good at helping to repair nerves, providing a anti-inflammatory, helping treat pancreatitis, helping treat hemorrhoids, and even helping treat osteoporosis. Generally anything that has to do with an inflammatory disease this mushroom has it covered.

Cordyceps

This is another mushroom that pretty much handled everything from sleeping patterns to appetite control and even helping to increase the overall stamina of a person. The funny part about this mushroom is that this mushroom begin giving us it's beneficial properties after we recognized that anything that we ate that ate it became stronger.

### *Mushrooms - Temperate Climates 40/70 Deg F*

Turkey Tail

This mushroom is already being used by the Japanese to treat a lot of different cancers in both preventing cancer as well as treating cancer. In addition to this, it does help reduce tumors and it also helps cure the Hepatitis B virus. Unlike some of the other mushrooms on this list, this mushroom can also help fight malaria.

## King Oyster

This mushroom helps to improve the overall stamina of a person and provide them with a load of antioxidants. Along with this, it can help improve blood levels in an individual especially if they are suffering from anemia. It does help with cholesterol levels as well.

## Mesima

This is another do it all type of mushroom since it can help with type 2 diabetes, hemorrhaging, increasing the immune system, providing antibacterial properties, helping with irritable bowel syndrome, and can even help with people who need to take laxatives. I think I'm beginning to like how many all-around mushrooms there are in the Mushroom Kingdom, are you?

## Cauliflower

This mushroom does something that the other mushrooms kind of do but this one specifically focuses on it. This mushroom helps fight skin diseases. It also helps fight issues causing anemia and can help fight against tumors. Just as well, this mushroom does have antifungal properties to it.

Chestnut

The reason why the chestnut mushroom is so important even though it has cousins that can be confused with the safer part of the chestnut mushroom family is that the big companies like  Advil, Tylenol and the other pain killer companies tend to use this as they're painkiller. That's right, this is the plant that they take from in order to give to you to treat that pain. It's also got some anti-cancer properties and can help with osteoporosis.

## Conclusion

Welcome to the end of this book and while I may have gone over it at least twice, or even thrice, I still want to bore this into you as much as possible because it is one of the crucial elements to surviving off of mushrooms if that is something you have to do. Do not consume anything unless you are 100% certain of what it is and you can identify all the notable marks of the mushroom itself. Do not trust anything else because it could be something that was a psychotropic, which would be bad in a survival situation, or it could be a poisonous plant, either way it's best just to avoid it if you don't know what it is and this is absolutely vital to understand. With that said I really hope you did enjoy this book and I'll see you next time.

# FREE Bonus Reminder

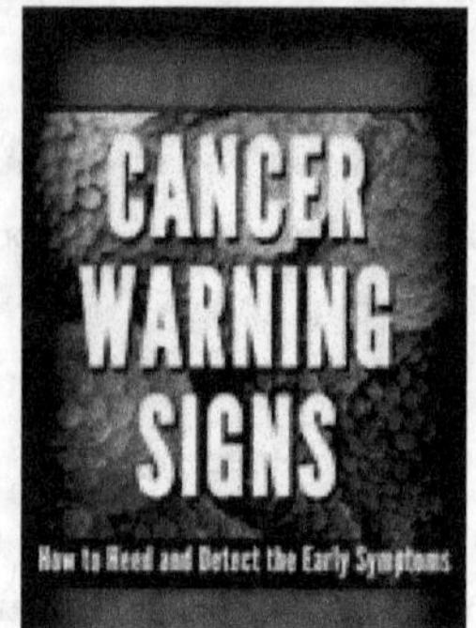

If you have not grabbed it yet, please go ahead and download your special bonus report *"Cancer Warning Signs. How To Heed & Detect The Early Symptoms!"*

Simply Click the Button Below

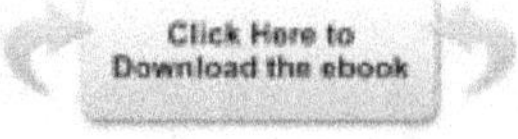


OR **Go to This Page**

http://healthylivingpeople.com/free/

## BONUS #2: More Free & Discounted Books or Products

**Do you want to receive more Free/Discounted Books or Products?**

We have a mailing list where we send out our new Books or Products when they go free or with a discount on Amazon. Click on the link below to sign up for Free & Discount Book & Product Promotions.

**=> Sign Up for Free & Discount Book & Product Promotions <=**

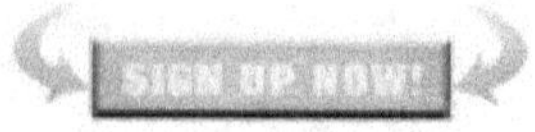

OR Go to this URL

**http://zbit.ly/1WBb1Ek**